My Journey of Hope

A Child's Guidebook for Living with Cancer

Sarah Jean Kovar

Foreword by Diane M. Komp

Illustrations by Barbara J. Hranilovich

ZondervanPublishingHouse
Grand Rapids, Michigan

A Division of HarperCollinsPublishers

Foreword
by Diane M. Komp, M.D.

This is a book that every adult should read.
Why?
Simply because it was written by a gentle teacher,
Written by a child, about an experience that
Few children, but many adults, will face.
Cancer.

You will not see a book like this
Published by a major publishing house very often.
Mostly, they deal with adult authors.
Mostly, adults wouldn't share thoughts and feelings
About life and death with strangers.
Mostly, adults wouldn't believe everything
That another adult had to say
About the thing that they fear the most.
Mostly, adults fear cancer.

But this was written by a child.
She tells us how she handles fear.

As young as she was, she knew that we,
Other kids, and adults too,
Need to hear the truth,
That the most important things for someone,
Young or old, with cancer are
Faith and hope.
"Trust me," she says.
And I do.

I've met hundreds of children like her,
Short on hair but long on wisdom.
For 25 years they've been my patients.
I would trust them with my life.
"It will be hard going through life with cancer,"
She admits,
"But it will be even tougher to get through
Without hope and faith."
Children who've outlived cancer
And those now with God will say the same.
Trust them.
They're right.

She talks to Jesus,
Hands her thoughts over to God.

"God did not make life fair," she says.
She knows the way that adults think.
If life doesn't turn out the way we want,
We blame it on God and then insist,
If that's the way it's going to be,
That there is no God
Or Sarah Jean would not even know
How to spell cancer.

But she spells it perfectly
And makes me wonder if my hand
Would not tremble more
Were this my book, not hers.
It is the Sarah Jeans that I will seek
When I must learn to spell.
It is her words "I continue to fight for my life"
That I will repeat.
Why don't you?

> —Diane M. Komp, M.D.
> author of *A Window to Heaven:*
> *When Children See Life in Death*

A Note from the Family

Early one morning, two hours before sunrise, Sarah Kovar, after waking frequently and feeling uneasy, asked her mother, Linda, to call Sister Kathleen, her dear friend.

"I'm scared," Sarah told her when she arrived.

Sister Kathleen gently took her hand and said, "Sarah, don't be afraid. The angels are waiting to welcome you, and you'll soon see Jesus. When you go home, please remember us."

Sarah responded, "I'll always hold all of you in my heart." Linda then left the room to get Sarah's father.

Sarah fought bravely with hope, while her parents, her little brother, Jason, other family members, and Sister Kathleen kept vigil with her through her few remaining days.

Sarah's deep faith in her Native American tradition and Catholic beliefs were an inspiration to all around her. Her Indian name was Mountain Woman Who

Speaks In Thunder, a name that suited her well, for she loved the mountains, which gave her peace and strength, and she also had the gift of speaking in tongues.

Sister Kathleen and Sarah shared a special bond. Sarah loved to talk to her special friend about the wonders of the Creator, and Sister Kathleen gave Sarah much support through her three-year battle with cancer. Sister Kathleen belongs to the Dominican Sisters of Sparkill, New York, and has worked with Native Americans since 1973 and continues this work in Great Falls, Montana, Sarah's hometown. One of Sister Kathleen's given Indian names is Angel Woman. Along with the name comes a Native American song, the Angel Spirit Song, which Sister Kathleen and other family members would sing to help Sarah during her final days.

Sarah began writing about her experiences with cancer two months after the removal of her first brain tumor, hoping to help other children deal with serious illness. A few days before Sarah died, Linda and Sister Kathleen completed the handmade version of this book. Sarah approved. Many believe that she resolved to stay alive until the book was completed, her gift of love to other children.

Sister Kathleen drew the original pictures according to Sarah's wishes and instructions, and the artist who redrew the pictures for this published version has followed the spirit of those originals closely. On the next page is Sister Kathleen's illustration of an eagle feather, similar to the one given to Sarah by her grandmother when she was a small child. This eagle feather is a sign of wisdom and courage. Sarah has truly earned this sacred symbol.

Sarah,
You have earned
an Eagle Feather
by your Courage –

*To all who helped me make it possible,
especially Sister Kathleen Kane.*

My Journey of Hope

Introduction

Hi, boys and girls. My name is Sarah Kovar and I have cancer. And because I have cancer, I have no hair. I can't do a lot of the things I could do before, like roller-skate, play baseball, and play basketball. But there's still much I can do. Sure, lots of things in life aren't fair, but you see, God did not make life fair.

In third grade, my grades started to drop; I was getting daydreamy and kept getting what we thought was flu. It turned out they were small seizures, signs of epilepsy, so the doctor set a time for me to have an EEG. That indicated I had some abnormal brain waves. So that led to surgery. And that meant a stay at the hospital. But after a while I handed my problem to the Lord and was able to sleep.

The reason I'm writing this book is to share my experiences with you. So if this ever happens to you, you will know what to expect.

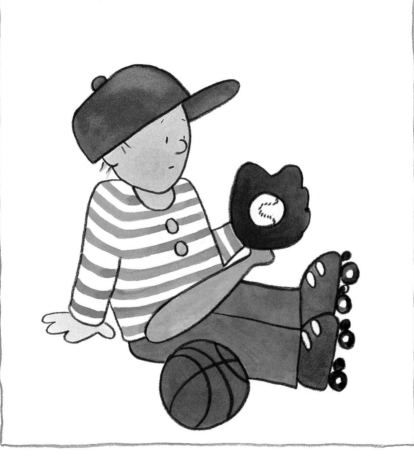

Surgery

The day before my surgery, a nurse told me about the two choices I had: a shot that would put me in a deep sleep or a gas mask that would do the same thing. I chose the mask. The next morning at 8:30 they got me ready for my operation. First the doctors shaved my head. Then they took me to a room that was the last room before the surgery room. This is where they put me to sleep. The surgery took 13 hours. After that I went to the recovery room. That's where you wake up from surgery. After that you go to I.C.U. The most I had to stay is two or three days. Then you are moved to a regular room. I bet you're wondering if there is a certain bedtime. Well, that's sort of up to you. If you want to get out quickly, you would want to go to bed about 9:00. Now if you want to stay there a while, you can go to bed any time you want. But the more you sleep, the faster your body will heal.

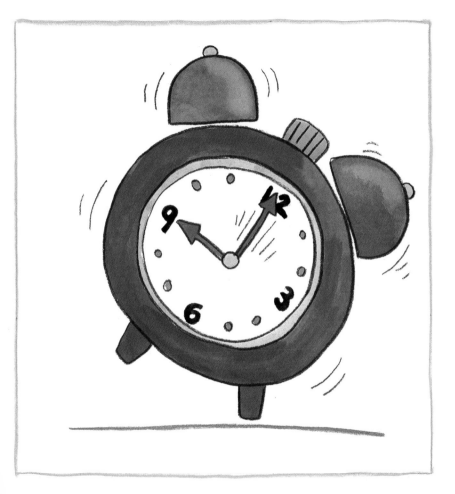

Treatment

Treatment can vary from just radiation to both chemo and radiation. You may not realize this: you might lose your hair. But it will grow back. You just have to be patient.

Radiation is ultraviolet rays. It kills fast-growing cells. So it kills the hair follicles. Some side effects are hair loss, nausea, and vomiting. You might get a little brown where you're being treated. Radiation is simple. All you do is lay on a table, and a laser beam goes on on either side of you.

Chemo is a little more difficult. You get poked. The side effects depend on what drugs you'll be taking. For instance, if you take Vincristine, you might get very sick to your stomach. There are pills to help you deal with these pains. Some drugs must be given in an overnighter at the hospital. I've had both kinds. In fact, I'm still taking the chemo that requires a stay at the hospital. You see, sometimes the therapy doesn't get all of the cancer cells so you have to get a different kind of chemotherapy.

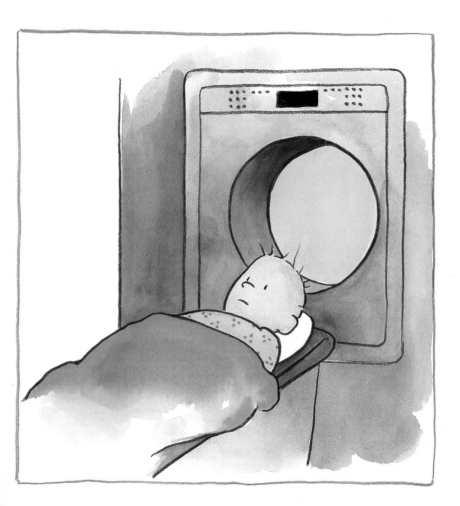

Blood Tests

In the course of the chemo, you will find that the doctors want a lot of blood tests. This is because they want to see how healthy it is. And also to see how the different types of blood cells are handling the treatment. Sometimes certain blood cells get low on their count so you have to get what is called a blood transfusion. A blood transfusion is where they match up your blood with a donor's blood. Once they get your blood matched, they put it in an IV bag. They connect the bag to the pole. Then they start the monitor. That controls how much blood is going into you at a time. It depends on how much blood you need to determine how long it will take. If you only need to get a unit of blood, it should only take 4 hours. They check your vital signs every 15 minutes. If you need help and your parents are not there, you can push the nurse button.

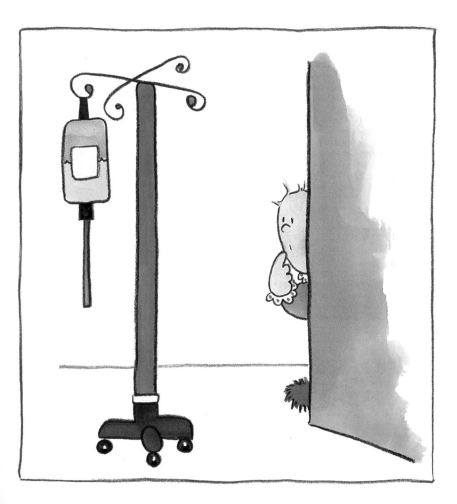

Hair Loss

Hair loss can be very hard to overcome. The thought of being bald—it is horrifying. But for all those who hate brushing and washing their hair, it is an advantage. One good thing about being bald is that it keeps you cool in the hot summer. If you are a girl, some people will mistake you for a boy. Some little kids might not understand why you are wearing a hat or why you do not have any hair. They may think it is funny and tease you. The best way to deal with it is to just ignore them. Believe me, it is no use to argue with them. If you feel uncomfortable about wearing hats and scarves but you do not want to go around without one of these on your head, you can look into buying a wig. When I lost my hair, I just accepted it. After a while, you will start to miss your hair. But really, there is nothing you or I can do about it. So we just have to be patient.

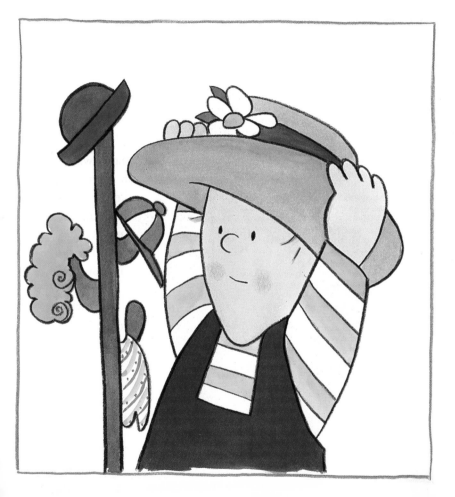

The Hospital Bed

Now since you will most likely be having a few stays at the hospital, I better tell you about the bed. It is designed to make you as comfortable as possible. You can raise the head of your bed if you get tired of lying down. You can also raise and lower the position of your feet and legs. If you want to watch television, there is a button on your bed that will turn it on for you and let you check the channels. And there is one last button near the bed. That is the nurse button. You use this for many reasons. Like if you throw up, you push it and a nurse will come and measure it and dump it. Or if you have an IV and you need to go to the bathroom, you just push it and she will help you. Or if you do not feel good, push it and the nurse will see what she can do about it. That is about all you need to know about the hospital bed.

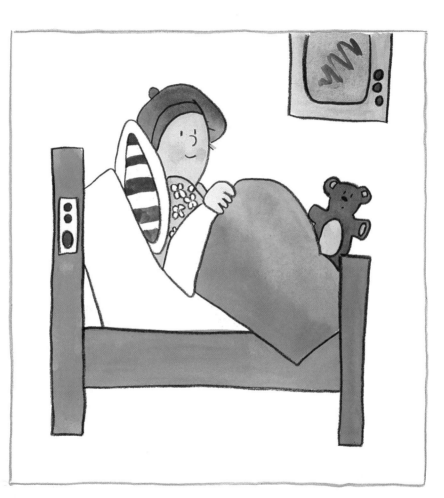

Hospital Entertainment

If you get bored of reading, writing, and watching television, there is a playroom that has games and puzzles. But if you do not want to do those things, there is a Nintendo that you are allowed to play for an hour. And if you still do not want to play the Nintendo, there is a VCR if you want to watch a movie. If you feel good enough, you can visit with a kid in another room. In a couple of days in the hospital, you can make a lot of friends and you can have a lot of fun.

So next time you have to go in, just think of how much fun you will have while you are there.

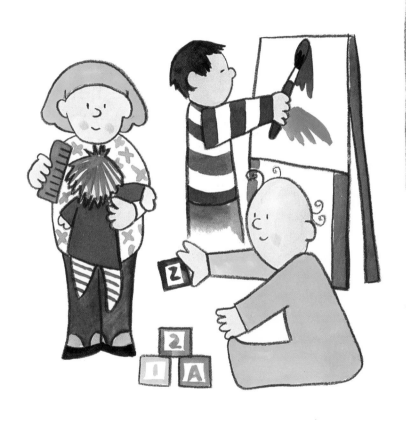

Bad Mood Swings

Once you start your treatment, you will find that you dislike going to the clinic or hospital. You may start to have bad moods when these days come. You might go to bed at 8:00 or 8:30, and you can sleep in till 10:00 but you still will be in a bad mood. When we learned that I had another tumor after the first treatment, every time we had to go to the clinic or hospital we were at each other's throats. And then when we got in the car, we would laugh about it.

One day we got a call that was an unexpected call for me to go in for my chemo. For the past few times we have not gotten upset. So one of the ways to keep you and your mom's throat in place, try not to think about the time of your appointment until the time comes.

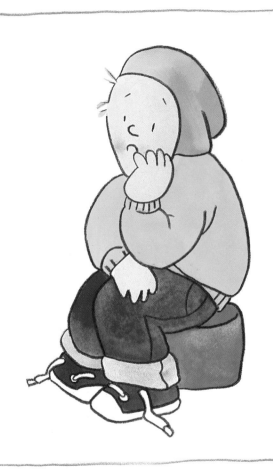

Hope and Faith

Two things you need to get through all the things that happen in the course of having cancer are faith and hope. Trust me, it will be hard going through life with cancer. But it will be even tougher to get through without hope and faith. In fact, those are the two things I depend on the most. When I learned that a tumor had started to grow again, I thought I would never be able to get through life. But I knew that I had to have faith in the Lord. So as I did before, I handed my thoughts to the Lord. I have to admit sometimes, I start to wonder if he's really helping me. Then my mom reminds me of the things he has done for me. Then I realize that he really is helping me. So if you start to feel run-down, think of the Lord and of all the things he is doing and all he has done to help you.

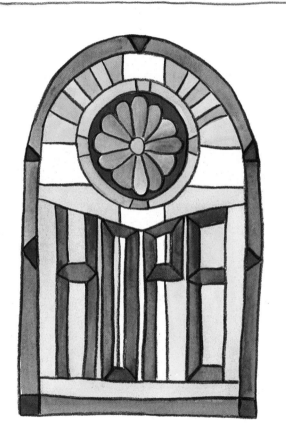

The Chinese Dinner

When I was done with the first year of chemotherapy, my mom and I went out to dinner. We were so glad because we thought it was the end of chemo for my life. We had dinner at 3-Ds restaurant. I had on a purple velvet dress with anklets and black dress shoes on. It was a delicious dinner. We sat in a family booth. I sat on one side and mom sat on the other. We had wonton soup and a special. After that, we picked up Jason's baby-sitter and took her home. We visited there a while. We went home and I was very happy when I went to bed that night.

Things were great for about four days. I was sitting on these steps. Mom told me that I had to have another surgery. But what I am trying to tell you is that you can have a good time even though you have cancer.

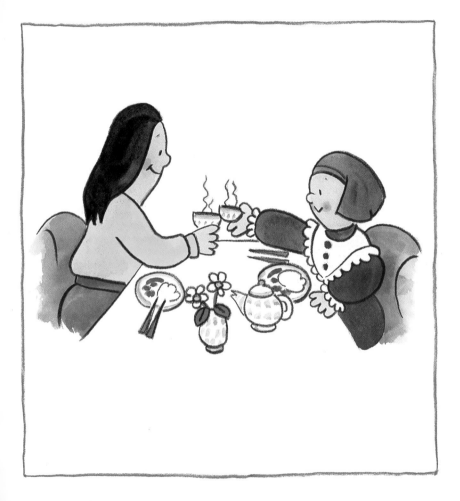

Seattle

I had my second surgery at the Children's Hospital in Seattle. It was a long trip. We left at 6:00 A.M. and we got there at 8:00 P.M. We stayed at Ronald McDonald House.

The Children's Hospital is a really big place. After I had my surgery, I was in for a week. Then they checked me over. They decided that I could have a weekend pass. My mom had to check my temperature every 8 hours. We had fun. On the first day we went on a ferry boat ride. The next few days we went to a place each day. I went back and got a portacal in. After that we went back to the Ronald McDonald House. A few days later we went home.

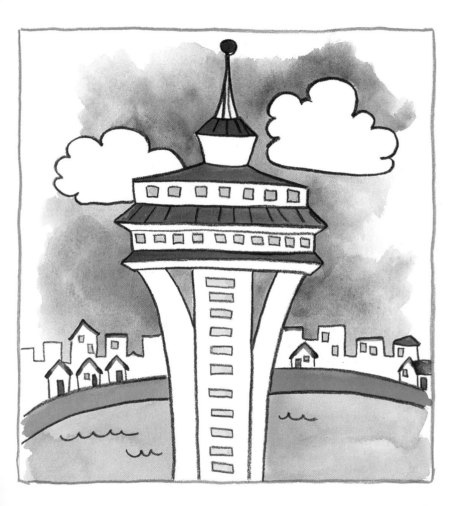

Accessories

There are some things in having cancer that you might need. One of these things is a port. A port is a little round metal ball with a rubber center. This port is useful if your veins are very tiny or bruised up. It is inserted near a large vein. Another thing is a feeding tube. It depends on how good you can keep your food down to decide what kind of tube you will have. You see, there are two kinds of tubes. One is G tube and one is a J tube. I have both the port and feeding tube. I have the G tube.

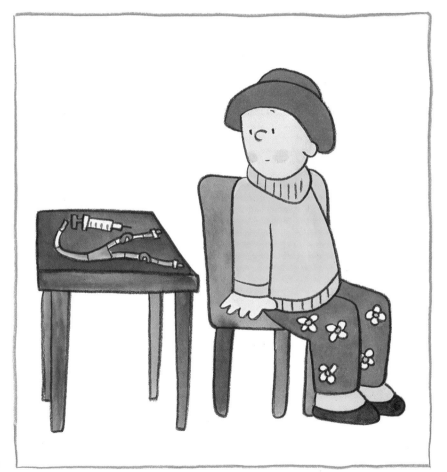

Sharing Feelings

There will be times you might feel upset or angry with yourself. It is important to share these feelings with someone. There are many people that you can share them with. One person I talk with is my mom. One other person I talk to is Jesus. You will discover after you talk over your feelings you feel much better.

Sometimes I cry. After I cry I feel better. When you start to feel that way, don't be afraid to let it out. If your parents won't listen, don't give up. Try looking into getting a counselor. Or try to get into a group that can help you.

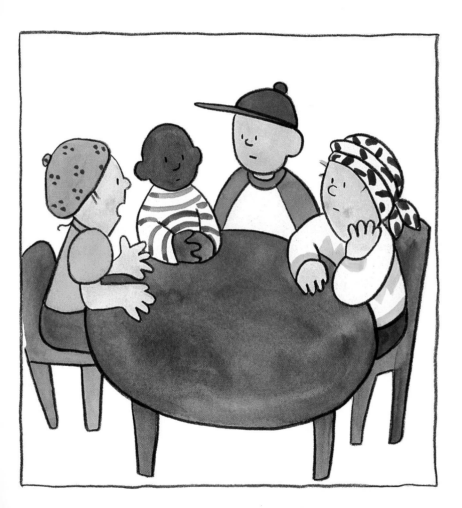

Rest

You will often find you get tired easily. This is a normal side effect. So if you are invited to a sleepover, tell your friends not to expect you to stay up as late as they do. It is important for you to get this rest. If you get tired at school, ask your teacher to call your mom. If the teacher says yes, call your mom and tell her you want to go home and rest. Do not be ashamed that you are taking naps. You are helping your body.

When you sleep, you also are restoring your body's energy. So when you get up from the nap you can have a lot of fun.

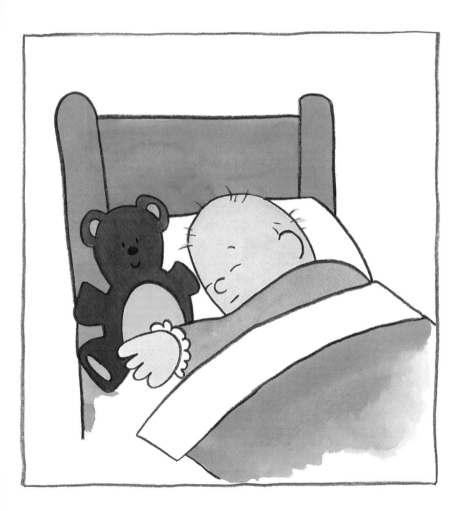

Hope Project Camp

The Highway Patrol put on a program called Hope. The way the program works is they ask you if you want anything, and give you a form. You therefore fill out the form and they will do what they can.

Every year for the past 6 years they have a camp by Glacier National Park in Montana. This year was the first time that I had been there. They did something every day. Here are the things that I did: I went to a chocolate factory on the first day. On the second day I went on an old-time tour bus up to the loop of the mountain. Then I went on an hour boat tour of Lake McDonald. On the last day of camp, I went on a helicopter ride. Then we went back to where we were staying, packed up, said our goodbyes, and went home.

So if you get picked by Project Hope, that is what to expect.

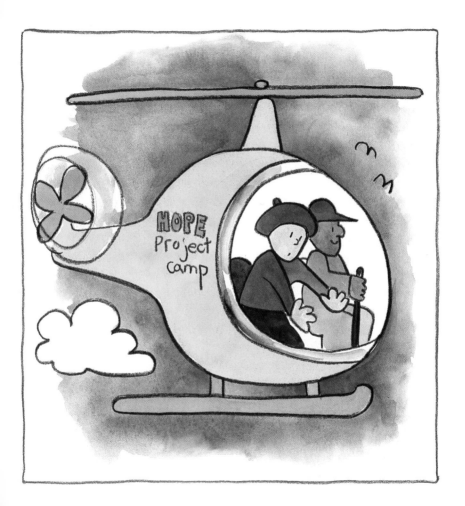

Death

In these chapters, I have shared with you what has happened to me and how I handled it. Well, here is my final chapter.

Cancer is a killer. It is a very sad thing, but true. It has now taken two of my very good, good friends. There are many good things about dying though. They are not suffering. They were lucky people. We are lucky people because we can be treated with the drugs we need. Some people can't. There are support groups if the grief gets too bad.

I plan to continue to fight for my life. Why don't you?

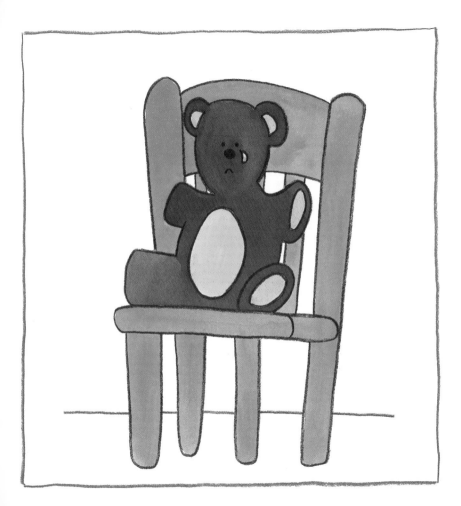

Who Are You?

(To Mr. Biscup, the best homeroom teacher yet.)
by Sarah Kovar

I walk quietly
amongst the
leaves and trees.
Who are you?
ask the leaves.
The trees ask,
Who are you?

I tell them
very quietly
I am Sarah
Kovar. I am
gentle.

I do not
have any
intention
to hurt you.

This is who I am.

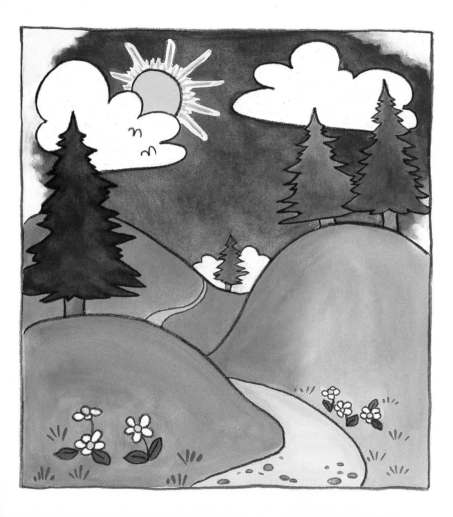

Hope

by Sarah Kovar

Without Hope
it is like living
in a dungeon
without any window.

With Hope
it is like
living in a
house with
three hundred windows.

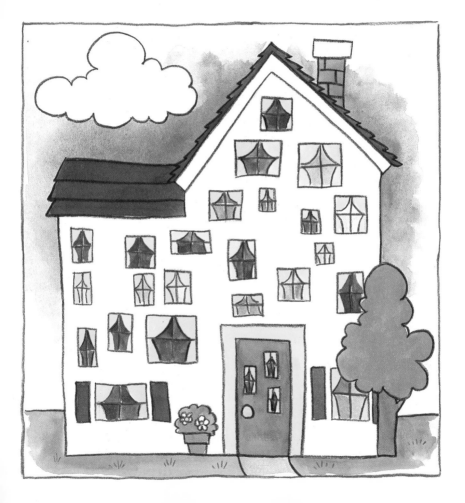

Requests for information should be addressed to:
Zondervan Publishing House
Grand Rapids, Michigan 49530

Library of Congress Cataloging-in-Publication Data

Kovar, Sarah Jean.
My journey of hope : a child's guidebook for living with cancer /
by Sarah Jean Kovar.
p.   cm.
ISBN 0-310-37450-2 (acid-free paper)
1. Tumors in children—Juvenile literature. I. Title.
RC281.C4K68   1993
362.1'9892994—dc20   93-7591
                                                CIP

Cover design and illustration by Barbara J. Hranilovich
Interior design by Bob Hudson and Florence Chambers
Typesetting by Nancy Wilson

Printed in the United States of America

93 94 95 96 97 98 99 00 01 / BP / 10 9 8 7 6 5 4 3 2 1

This edition is printed on acid-free paper and meets
the American National Standards Institute Z39.48 standard.